# Infectious Disease:

# Fast Focus Study Guide

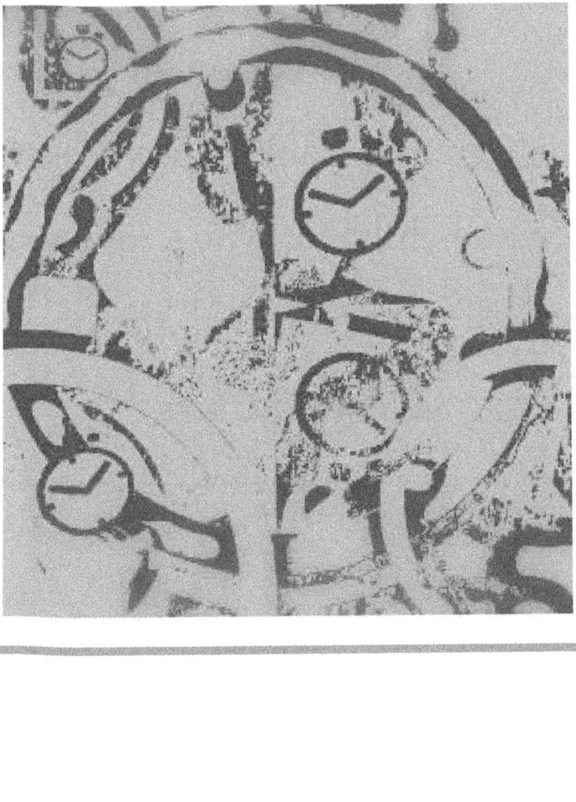

Acknowledgements

I dedicate this book to my beautiful wife and children, who I love more than all the water in all the oceans and all the seas.

CONTENTS

- This book is written for any medical professionals who want to learn more about Infectious Disease.

- There are over 350 pages of easy to read facts about Infectious Disease.

- Put this book in your bathroom or on your coffee table.

- This is the perfect graduation gift for the aspiring physician or graduating physician.

- This Fast Focus Study Guide will provide you with a practical review of the key information you need to know.

- Buy this book now if you want this quick and concise information

**Can Actinomyces be diagnosed by isolation of Actinomyces from an asymptomatic patient?**

No, patients must by symptomatic

**Is there an association between intrauterine devices (IUD) and pelvic actinomycosis?**

Yes

**What are within Actinomyces sulfur granules?**

The sulfur granules are actually nests of the Actinomyces bacteria

**What conditions are associated with abdominal actinomycosis?**

It occurs most frequently after bowel perforation, bowel surgery, and diverticulitis

**What is the most common location of abdominal actinomycosis?**

Abdominal actinomycosis occurs most frequently at the Ileocecal valve

**Which disease is associated with isolation of "sulfur granules" from a draining infection?**

Actinomycosis

**What at the characteristic findings of Actinomycosis?**

This disease is characterized by gram positive branching organisms and sulfur granules

**What is the mechanism of Acyclovir?**

This drug inhibits viral DNA polymerases after phosphorylation by viral thymidine kinase

**How does acyclovir work against HSV-I and HSV-II infections?**

Orally absorbed and activated by HSV thymidine kinase, it interferes with production of new viruses

**What is the etiology of African sleeping sickness?**

Trypanosoma brucei (transmitted by the tsetse fly)

**Which disease is characterized by a hypersensitivity reaction to Aspergillus?**

Allergic Broncho pulmonary aspergillosis

**Which drug is used prophylactically for influenza A and rubella? It works by blocking the viral penetration?**

Amantadine

**What is the mechanism of Aminoglycosides?**

Aminoglycosides inhibit the binding of 50s to 30s and causes misreading of mRNA. Aminoglycosides require O2 for uptake and is ineffective against anaerobes

**What are the common toxicities of Amphotericin B?**

Azotemia; Anemia; Hypokalemia; Nausea; Anorexia; Phlebitis; Hypomagnesaemia

**What is the mechanism of Amphotericin B?**

Amphotericin B binds to ergosterol and forms membrane pores that disrupt homeostasis

**What are the common gram negative anaerobic bacteria?**

Bacteroides, Prevotella, Porphyromonas, and Fusobacterium

**What are the most common gram positive anaerobic cocci bacteria?**

Peptostreptococcus and anaerobic Streptococcus

**What is wool sorters disease?**

Pulmonic bacillus anthrax

**What is the most common cause of viral aseptic meningitis?**

Enterovirus

**What is the most common cause of Aspergillus infection?**

Aspergillus fumigatus

**What is the most common predisposing factor to the development of invasive aspergillosis?**

Prolonged neutropenia from cytotoxic chemotherapy or leukemia

**What is the probable etiology of a sputum with branching septate hyphae in an immunocompromised patient?**

This is most likely to be Aspergillus species

**Is there an increased risk of babesiosis after splenectomy?**

Yes

**How often are people co-infected with Babesia microti and Borrelia burgdorferi (Lyme disease)?**

Approximately 10% of patients are co-infected

**What is the incubation period for babesiosis?**

The incubation period is approximately 1-4 weeks

**What is the peak incidence of babesiosis?**

Babesiosis has a peak incidence from May to September

**What is the vector for the genus Babesia?**

The deer tick (Ixodes scapularis)

**What state has the highest number of reported cases of babesiosis?**

New York State

**Which two types of Babesia are responsible for most human infections?**

Babesia microti and Babesia divergens

**Which type of Babesia is associated with the most severe form of the disease?**

Babesia divergens is associated with a most severe illness

**How often do patients with non-gonococcal bacterial arthritis have only a single joint involved?**

Approximately 80% of the time only a single joint will be involve

**What are the typical findings of gonococcal bacterial arthritis?**

These patients generally have a migratory arthritis and pustules of the trunk and extremities

**What is the hallmark of a non-gonococcal infectious bacterial arthritis?**

Acute onset of a single swollen painful joint

**What is the most common non-gonococcal cause of bacterial arthritis?**

Staphylococcus aureus

## What is BCG?

BCG (Bacillus Calmette-Guerin) is a live attenuated strain of mycobacterium bovis used in some countries

**Do dog bite wounds have a higher infection rate than human bite wounds?**

No, human bite wounds have a higher infection rate (20%) than dog bite wounds (5%)

**What is the most common bacteria to cause infections within 24 hours of a cat bite?**

Pasteurella multocida and Pasteurella septica

**Which bite wounds have the highest infection rate?**

Cat bite wounds have the highest infection rate (approximately 20-40%)

**What is the most common extra pulmonary manifestation of blastomycosis?**

Cutaneous lesions are the most common extra pulmonary manifestation of blastomycosis

**What is the most common genitourinary manifestation of blastomycosis?**

Infection of the prostate is the most common GU manifestation of blastomycosis

**What are the three types of botulism?**

Food borne disease; Infant botulism;
Wound botulism

**Describe the gram stain of Clostridium botulinum?**

Clostridium botulinum is a gram positive, anaerobic bacteria

**How long does it take for symptoms to develop after ingestion of botulinum toxin?**

12-36 hours

**What are the three common manifestations of botulism?**

Food-borne botulism, infant botulism, and wound botulism

**What determines the severity of food-borne botulism?**

The severity of botulism is determined by the amount of toxin ingested

**What is the most common cause of food-borne botulism?**

Poorly prepared home canned foods

**How often do patients presenting with a brain abscess have papilledema?**

About 25% of patients will have papilledema

**How often does hematogenous spread of infection from a distant site account for brain abscesses?**

This occurs in approximately 25% of brain abscesses

**What is the classic triad of patients presenting with a brain abscess?**

Headache

Fever

Focal neurological deficit

**What is the most common presenting symptom for patients with a brain abscess?**

Approximately 70% of patients will present with a non-localizing headache

**Which disease is seen in abattoir workers?**

Brucellosis

**What causes approximately 90% of infectious bursitis?**

Staph aureus

**How often will patients with disseminated candidiasis have negative blood cultures?**

Approximately 50% of patients could have negative blood cultures

**What specific organism is the most common cause of candidemia?**

Candida albicans

**Which infection is associated with cotton wool patches on retinal exam?**

Disseminated candidiasis

**What are two antibiotics appropriate for outpatient management of cat and dog bites?**

Amoxicillin-Clavulanate (Augmentin)

Penicillin

(Remember to give the tetanus toxoid to update vaccination)

**What is the most common etiology of catheter related bacteremia?**

Staphylococcus epidermidis

**Which disorder is characterized by regional lymphadenopathy within 2 weeks of exposure to a cat scratch?**

Cat-scratch disease secondary to Bartonella henselae infection

**Describe the mechanism of cephalosporin antibiotics?**

Cephalosporin antibiotics are bactericidal beta-lactam drugs that inhibit cell wall synthesis

**Transmission of this parasite occurs via the bite of reduviid bug?**

Trapanosoma cruzi (Chagas's disease)

**What organ is most commonly involved with Chagas's disease?**

The heart is the organ most commonly involved with Chagas's disease

**Is it true that clinical infection with chancroid (Haemophilus ducrey) is uncommon in women?**

Yes

**What are the typical physical exam findings in patients with chancroid?**

Painful genital ulceration and tender inguinal adenopathy

**What will the gram stain of a cultured base in a patient with Chancroid (Haemophilus ducreyi)?**

The gram stain of the ulcer exudate will be significant for gram negative coccobacilli in a "school of fish"

**Which STD is caused by Ducrey's bacillus? The skin lesion occurs 2-4 days after exposure?**

Chancroid

**How long are people infectious during their illness with chickenpox?**

People are infectious from 2 days prior to onset of symptoms until all of the lesions develop crusts

**What is the incubation period for chickenpox?**

The incubation period for chickenpox is approximately 9-21 days

**What is the virus responsible for chickenpox?**

Varicella-Zoster

**When during the year is the peak time for chickenpox?**

The peak incidence for chickenpox is in the spring

**How often do gonococcal infections occur concomitantly with chlamydia infection?**

Approximately 45% of gonococcal infection occurs concomitantly with chlamydial infection

**Name two symptoms in patients with mucopurulent cervicitis secondary to chlamydial infection?**

Vaginal discharge

Spotting after intercourse

**What are the typical findings of a vaginal infection with Chlamydia trachomatis?**

Mucopurulent cervicitis

Vaginal discharge

Sometimes with friable cervix

Numerous WBC with no clue cells, no yeast, no trichomonads

**What is the drug of choice for treating of chlamydial infection in pregnant women?**

Erythromycin

**What is the most common cause of sexually transmitted disease in the US?**

Chlamydia trachomatis

**What is the most common reportable infection in the US?**

Chlamydia trachomatis

**What is the mechanism of chloramphenicol?**

Chloramphenicol is bacteriostatic by inhibiting the 50S peptidyl transferase

**What is the mechanism of fluoroquinalones like ciprofloxacin and levofloxacin?**

Inhibits DNA gyrase (topoisomerase III)

**Which bacteria are treated with clindamycin?**

Anaerobes

**What is the relapse rate of Clostridium difficile and what is the treatment of relapse?**

The relapse rate is about 20% and the treatment is the same.

**What is the most common opportunistic infection of the nervous system in patients with AIDS?**

CMV

**Which fungus is known to cause arthritis, also known as desert rheumatism?**

Coccidioides immitis

**Which fungus spores are found in the desert southwest and are known to cause valley fever?**

Coccidioides immitus

**Which cause of endocarditis is strongly linked with colon cancer?**

Streptococcus bovis

**How often do the sexual partners of patients with condyloma acuminatum develop the disease?**

Approximately 40-60% of sexual partners will contract condyloma acuminatum from their infected

**What are the soft flesh colored papular or pedunculated lesions caused by HPV?**

Condyloma acuminatum

**Which types of HPV are generally associated with exophytic warts?**

HPV 6 and 11

**Which types of HPV are generally associated with flat warts?**

HPV 16 and 18

**Which bacteria has a gram stain showing club shaped organisms that look like "Chinese letters"?**

Corynebacterium diptheriae

**What is the most common presentation for patients with cryptococcosis?**

Meningitis (>90% of patients)

**What is the classic stain used to identify Cryptococcus neoformans?**

India ink stain

**What is the sensitivity of the India ink stain of the CSF in the diagnosis of cryptococcal meningitis?**

60-80%

**Which disease is characterized as encapsulated yeast on India ink preparation of cerebral spinal fluid?**

Cryptococcus neoformans

**What are the most common presenting symptom in patients with cryptosporidium parvum?**

Diarrhea

**What is the most common cause of waterborne diarrhea in the US?**

Giardia lamblia

**What is the most common cause of Campylobacter enteritis?**

Campylobacter jejuni is the most common cause of Campylobacter enteritis.

**What is the most common clinical presentation of diphtheria?**

Sore throat and malaise

**Describe the atypical lymphocytes of EBV (mono)?**

Suppressor/Cytotoxic T-Cells that suppress B-cell proliferation and immunoglobulin production and are cytotoxic to the EBV infected B Cells

**If the mono spot test for EBV is negative and infection is suspected, which 3 tests could be ordered?**

Anti- early

Anti-viral capsid

Anti EBV nuclear antigens

**What are the most common symptoms at presentation in patients with empyema?**

Cough, fever, chest pain, dyspnea

**What is the most common cause of empyema?**

Staphylococcus aureus

**Which type of infection is most commonly responsible for empyema?**

Anaerobic bacterial infections

**Which diseases predispose to infections with encapsulated organisms?**

Sickle cell disease

Asplenia

Agammaglobulinemia

**What is the most common arbovirus infection in the United States?**

Saint Louis encephalitis

**What is the most common cause of viral encephalitis diagnosed?**

Herpes simplex

**Which viral encephalitis is characterized by MRI findings of temporal lobe inflammation?**

Herpes simplex encephalitis

**Bacterial endocarditis with these two organisms have been associated with colon cancer?**

Streptococcus bovis

Clostridium septicus

**Describe the incidence of neurologic manifestations in patients with bacterial endocarditis?**

Approximately 1/3 of patients will develop neurologic symptoms.

**How often do Osler's nodes develop in patients with bacterial endocarditis?**

Osler's nodes are small tender nodules on the fingers and toes seen in 20-25% of patients with bacteria

**What are Janeway spots, seen in patents with bacterial endocarditis?**

Small non tender macules on the palms and soles

**What is the most common cause of death associated with endocarditis?**

Congestive heart failure related to aortic insufficiency

**What is the most common etiology of fungal endocarditis in IV drug users?**

Candida parapsilosis

**What is the organism most commonly responsible for prosthetic valve endocarditis?**

Coagulase negative staphylococcus

**What is the yield of a transthoracic echocardiogram (TTE) and a trans-esophageal echocardiogram (TEE) in the setting of native valve endocarditis?**

The TTE in native valve endocarditis will be positive in 50-80% of patients and the TEE will be diagnostic

**Which two heart valves are most commonly effected in endocarditis secondary to IV drug use?**

Aortic valve

Tricuspid valve

**Which heart valves are most commonly involved in candida endocarditis?**

The aortic and mitral valves are most commonly involved in candida endocarditis

**Which intestinal protozoan pathogen invades colonic epithelium and exerts cytopathic effect? It causes fever/bloody stools/cramping. Hepatic abscess may occur secondary to extra intestinal spread?**

Entamoeba histolytica

**What is the transmission of Entamoeba histolytica?**

Fecal oral

**What parasite is known to cause amebiasis?**

Entamoeba histolytica

**Where are most infections from Entamoeba histolytica localized?**

Large bowel

**What is the most common parasitic worm infection in the U.S.?**

Enterobius vermicularis

**What is the most common symptom of Enterobius vermicularis?**

Perianal pruritus

**What is the most common cause of epididymitis in young sexually active men?**

Neisseria gonorrhea and Chlamydia trachomatis

**What is the most common cause of epididymitis in men over 35 y/o?**

Gram negative aerobic rods

**What is St. Anthony's fire?**

Erysipelas-- superficial cellulitis of the skin and cutaneous lymphatics

**What is the most common etiology of erysipelas?**

Beta-hemolytic strep infection

**What is the cause of erythema infectiosum?**

Parvovirus B 19

**What is the typical rash of erythema infectiosum (parvovirus B-19)?**

Erythema infectiosum is associated with the classic "slapped cheek" rash

**Which infectious disease has been commonly associated with erythema multiforme?**

Herpes simplex infections

**What is a felon?**

A felon is a closed space infection of the distal phalanx

**What are the two parameters required for diagnosis of fever of unknown origin?**

Temperature >101.0

At least one week of intensive diagnostic evaluation

**Which bacterial causes non healing skin ulceration in people who work with fish tanks?**

Mycobacterium marinum

**What is Fournier's gangrene?**

Necrotizing fasciitis of the male or female genitalia

**What is the mechanism of ganciclovir?**

Phosphorylation by viral kinase preferentially inhibits CMV DNA polymerase

**Which group of bacteria are covered by Gentamycin?**

Gram negative bacteria

**Deficiency of intestinal IgA may cause susceptibility to this parasite?**

Giardia lamblia

**What is the most common symptom of intestinal giardiasis?**

Abdominal bloating

**What is the sensitivity of three stool samples in the workup of possible giardiasis?**

Three stool samples will have about a 90% sensitivity when attempting to make the diagnosis of giardia

**What is the etiology of a urethral or endocervical exudate with leukocytes containing gram negative bacteria?**

Neisseria gonorrhea infection

**What is the mechanism of griseofulvin?**

Griseofulvin interferes with microtubule function and disrupts mitosis

**What is the most common long term bacterial infection worldwide?**

Helicobacter pylori

**What are the five HACEK organisms?**

Haemophilus

Aggregatibacter

Cardiobacterium

Eikenella

Kingella

**Which animal is associated with spread of Hantavirus to humans?**

Deer mice

**Can Hepatitis A cross the placenta?**

Hepatitis A has not been shown to cross the placenta

**How is the diagnosis for acute hepatitis B made?**

Acute hepatitis B infection is diagnosed by the presence of IgM HBc Ab and HBs Ag

**How is the diagnosis of acute hepatitis A made?**

HAV-IgM

How is the diagnosis of acute hepatitis C made?

Detection of Anti HCV

**What are the first two lab abnormalities in acute hepatitis B infections?**

Elevated ALT

Development of Anti HBc

**What are the two diagnostic tests for acute hepatitis B?**

HBsAg (hepatitis B surface antigen;

Anti HBc-IgM

**What is the first marker for acute hepatitis B to show in the serum?**

First - Hepatitis B surface antigen

Second - IgM Anti-HBc

**What is the incubation period for Hepatitis A?**

The incubation period for Hepatitis A is 15-45 days

**What is the incubation period for Hepatitis B?**

The incubation period for Hepatitis B is 30-180 days

**What is the term for hepatitis D simultaneously infected with hepatitis B?**

Coinfection

**What percentage of people with hepatitis C develop anti-HCV?**

At 6 weeks approximately 70% of patients with hepatitis C infection will have anti HCV, and at 6 month

**Does hepatitis A cause cirrhosis or chronic hepatitis?**

No

**How are hepatitis A IgG antibodies interpreted?**

IgG anti hepatitis A antibodies are indicative of an infection with hepatitis A within the previous months

**How are hepatitis A IgM antibodies interpreted?**

IgM anti hepatitis A antibodies are indicative of a recent infection with hepatitis A

**How long does it take for an acute illness from hepatitis A to resolve?**

Acute illness from hepatitis A generally resolves in a period of 2-6 weeks

**How often does hepatitis A cause fulminant hepatitis?**

Approximately 1% of patients

**Are people with the anti-HBs antibody protected from infection with hepatitis B?**

Yes, the presence of the anti-HBs is a marker of immunity from hepatitis B

**Does the presence of HBe antigen indicate that the patient is infectious?**

Yes, the presence of the HBe antigen indicates that the patient is infectious

**How long does the HBe antigen generally seen in the blood of infected patients?**

The HBe antigen is generally detectable for 2-6 weeks

**How often will HBeAg positive mothers infect their newborns if no intervention is taken?**

Approximately 90% will infect their newborns with hepatitis B if no intervention is taken

**What does the presence of HBe antigen indicate?**

The HBe antigen in the blood indicates that hepatitis B is actively replicating

**What is indicated by a positive HBsAg?**

The presence of HBsAg indicates an acute or chronic infection with hepatitis B

**What is indicated by the presence of anti-HBc antibody in the serum?**

Anti-HBc antibody is an indication of previous infection with hepatitis B

**What is indicated by the presence of anti-HBc?**

Anti-HBc is the earliest indication of an acute infection

**What is indicated by the presence of anti-Hbe?**

Anti-Hbe indicates resolution of an acute infection with hepatitis B

**When is the HBs-Ag generally detectable after exposure to hepatitis B?**

The HBS-Ag generally is detectable at 1-4 months

**How long can it take for patients infected with hepatitis C to develop hepatitis C antibodies?**

It can take up to a year for some people infected with hepatitis C to develop hepatitis C antibodies

**How often will patients with hepatitis C develop chronic hepatitis?**

Approximately 80% of patients with hepatitis C will develop chronic hepatitis

**What is the most common cause of chronic viral hepatitis?**

Hepatitis C

**Does herpes simplex 1 generally infect the lips and perioral region and herpes simplex 2 genital region?**

Yes

**Can HSV-1 be associated with painful urination?**

Yes

**How is herpes simplex (HSV-1 and HSV-2) transmitted?**

Herpes simplex is transmitted through infected secretions

**How often are new herpes simplex 2 (HSV-2) infections symptomatic?**

Approximately 33% of new HSV-2 infections are symptomatic

**How often is herpes simplex 2 responsible for genital herpes infections?**

HSV-2 is responsible for 70-95% of the genital herpes infections

**How often will herpes simplex 1 of the lips or perioral region recur?**

Approximately 20-40% of primary herpes simplex 1 infections of the lips or perioral regions will recur.

**How often will herpes simplex 2 of the genital region recur?**

Approximately 60-80% of HSV-2 of the genital region will recur

**Are there a treatment for herpes infections?**

Yes, acyclovir, valacyclovir, or famciclovir can all be used to treat herpes infections.

**What is the incubation period for HSV-2 genital infections?**

The incubation period of HSV-2 is about 2-7 days

**What is the term given for a herpes infection of the finger?**

Herpes simplex 1 or herpes simplex 2 can infect the finger resulting in herpetic whitlow

**How often does HSV cutaneous dissemination occur in immunocompromised patients?**

Cutaneous dissemination occurs in approximately 1/3 of immunocompromised patients

**How often does HSV cutaneous dissemination occur in non-immunocompromised patients?**

Cutaneous dissemination is seen in approximately 2-4% of patients

**How often does herpes zoster occur in children?**

Approximately 10% of cases of herpes zoster occur in children

**How often does post herpetic neuralgia develop in patients with normal immune systems?**

Among this population, post herpetic neuralgia develops in about 10% of patients

**How often does recurrent zoster develop?**

Approximately 3-5% of patients will have a recurrence of zoster after an initial episode

**Is there a seasonal pattern to zoster (shingles)?**

No

**Is topical acyclovir used for the treatment of zoster?**

No

**Should you place hospitalized patients with zoster (shingles) into isolation?**

Yes, these patients should be placed in isolation

**What is the definition of post herpetic neuralgia in patients with a history of herpes zoster (shingles)?**

Pain that persists more than 30 days after onset of rash or after healing of the skin lesions

**What is the definition of post herpetic neuralgia?**

Pain persisting longer than 4-6 weeks after the appearance of the herpes zoster rash

**What is the etiology of the term shingles?**

Shingles is derived from the Latin word cingulum which means girdle

**What is the meaning of the word zoster?**

Zoster is a Greek word meaning belt

**What is the most common complication of herpes zoster?**

Post herpetic neuralgia

**What is the most common location of zoster (shingles)?**

Shingles most commonly occurs on the thorax

**What is the Ramsay-Hunt syndrome?**

Infection of the geniculate ganglion of the seventh cranial nerve is called the Ramsay-Hunt syndrome.

**What is the term given for herpes zoster infection involving the the first division of the trigeminal neuralgia?**

Herpes Zoster Ophthalmicus

**Which 3 drugs are approved in the US for the treatment of herpes zoster (shingles)?**

Acyclovir, valacyclovir, and famciclovir

**What is the classic radiographic findings of disseminated Histoplasmosis?**

Diffuse reticulonodular infiltrates

**What is the most common etiology of infectious lung granulomas?**

Histoplasmosis

**How much isoniazid therapy should be given for HIV positive patients with a positive PPD?**

A year of daily isoniazid chemoprophylaxis

**What is the differential diagnosis for cerebral mass in person with AIDS?**

Toxoplasmosis

Acute stroke

Metastatic Kaposi's sarcoma

Encephalitis

**What is the mechanism of AZT?**

Preferentially inhibits reverse transcriptase of HIV

**Can genital herpes be spread without contact with herpetic lesion?**

25% of infections are caused by contact with asymptomatic individual who is shedding HSV from the genital tract.

**What are six common herpes viruses which may infect humans?**

HSVI

HSVII

CMV

VZV

EBV

**What is the clinical difference between HSV I and HSV II genital infections?**

HSV II - more severe and recurrent genital tract infection

HSV I - mild and rapidly diminishing in frequency

**What is the difference between primary, initial, and recurrent genital herpes?**

Initial - first time person is infected

Primary - occurs in 1/3 of individuals without antibodies. It is widely spread lasting 12-21 days

Recurrent - lasts 2-4 days

**What is the most common cause of malabsorption in patients with IgA deficiency?**

Giardiasis

**How long does it generally take for infectious mononucleosis to run its course?**

Symptoms will resolve in 1-3 weeks in the majority of people

**Is infectious mononucleosis associated with changes in the hepatic enzymes?**

Approximately 60-90% of patients will develop abnormalities in the AST and ALT

**Is infectious mononucleosis associated with splenic rupture?**

Splenic rupture is not common but it has been described.

**Is the Epstein Barr Virus associate with any malignancies?**

Yes, EBV has been associated with Burkitt's lymphoma and nasopharyngeal carcinoma

**Is the Epstein Barr Virus common in our population?**

Yes, approximately 50% of the population in the US has serologic evidence of exposure by 5 y/o

**What are the common symptoms of infectious mononucleosis?**

The most common symptoms are fever, lymphadenopathy, and pharyngitis

**What are the neurologic complications of Epstein Barr virus?**

Less than 1% of patients develop neurologic complications of EBV.

**What changes in the CBC are common in the setting of infectious mononucleosis?**

Infectious mononucleosis is associated with a lymphocytosis with atypical lymphocytes.

**What is the mechanism of infectious mononucleosis associated hemolytic anemia?**

Patients can develop an autoantibody to the "i" antigen on the red cells

**What is the most common clinical manifestation of a primary EBV infection?**

Infectious mononucleosis

**What is the most common way that infectious mononucleosis is diagnosed?**

Patients are tested for the presence of heterophile antibodies by using tests such as the mono spot test

**What is the primary treatment for infectious mononucleosis?**

Patients should be monitored for complications of mononucleosis and should receive supportive care.

**What is the etiology of intestinal amebiasis?**

Entamoeba histolytica

**List four side effects of isoniazid?**

Peripheral neuropathy secondary to Vitamin B6 deficiency

Mood elevation, decreased appetite secondary to MAO inhibition

Elevated SGOT and bilirubin

Hepatitis

**What is the mechanism of INH?**

Decreases synthesis of mycolic acids

**Kala-azar is another name for visceral leishmaniasis, what is the etiology?**

Leishmania donovani

**What is the mechanism of ketoconazole?**

Ketoconazole functions by inhibiting ergosterol synthesis in susceptible fungi

**What are the common presenting findings in patients with Legionella?**

Purulent Sputum

Gram stain without organisms

Failure to respond to conventional antibiotics

Temperature-pulse dissociation with rapidly progressive pneumonia

Hyponatremia

**What is the most common cause of polyneuropathy in the world?**

Leprosy

**Are pregnant women at particular risk of developing Listeria?**

Yes, up to 1/3 of patients infected with Listeria are pregnant women

**Can Listeria cause endocarditis?**

Yes, Listeria can cause endocarditis, most often left sided, and often associated with systemic bacteria

**Can people be non-symptomatic carriers of Listeria?**

Yes, approximately 5% of people can be healthy carriers, with bacteria found in the rectum or vagina

**What is the annual incidence of Listeria meningitis in the US?**

The annual incidence of Listeria meningitis is approximately 9.7/100,000 people.

**What is the mortality of granulomatosis infantiseptica caused by Listeria infection?**

The mortality is approximately 33-100%

**What is the most common clinical manifestation of Listeria infections?**

Meningitis

**What is the most common early manifestation of perinatal Listeria infections?**

Chorioamnionitis

**What is the most common presentation of central nervous system infection in patients with Listeria?**

The most common CNS infection is meningitis

**What is the most common subtype of Leptospirosis interrogans?**

The canicola serogroup is the most common cause of leptospirosis in the US

**What is the only strain of Listeria bacteria to infect humans?**

Listeria monocytogenes

**When does Listeria monocytogenes infection most commonly occur in pregnancy?**

Listeria infection most commonly occurs during the third trimester of pregnancy

**Which bacteria are associated with tumbling motility when grown in saline suspensions?**

Listeria

**What is the most common cause of amoebic liver abscesses?**

Entameba histolytica reaches the liver via portal vein. Surgical drainage is contraindicated

**Which lobe of the liver is most likely to develop a liver abscess?**

The majority of liver abscesses are seen in the right lobe of the liver

**What is the etiology of Loeffler's pneumonia?**

Ascaris lumbricoides

**How often are lung abscesses associated with lung cancer in patients over 50 y/o?**

Approximately 30% of lung abscesses in this population will be associated with an underlying lung cancer

**Are there symptoms associated with the rash of erythema migrans?**

Often, but not always. People will experience malaise, fatigue, and low grade fever at the time they develop

**How long does the tick have to be attached before it is able to transmit Lyme disease?**

In general, the tick is attached for approximately 48 hours before it can transmit Lyme disease.

**How often do cardiac manifestations develop in patients with Lyme disease?**

Myocarditis is seen in approximately 8% of patients with untreated Lyme disease.

**How often do neurologic manifestations occur in patients with Lyme disease?**

Approximately 10% of untreated patients can develop neurologic symptoms.

**How often do patients presenting with Lyme disease actually remember the tick bite?**

Less than 50% of the patients diagnosed with Lyme disease will remember the tick bite.

**How often is the characteristic rash, erythema migrans, seen in patients with Lyme disease?**

It is estimated that only 50-75% of patients will develop noticeable erythema migrans.

**In patients who develop Lyme disease, when does the characteristic rash (erythema migrans) develop?**

Erythema migrans is seen 3-32 days (median 7 days) after the tick bite.

**What are the cardiac manifestations of Lyme disease?**

Heart block and mild myopericarditis are the typical cardiac manifestations of Lyme disease.

**What are the most common neurologic symptoms of Lyme disease?**

Headaches, mild stiff neck, and photophobia

**What is the causative agent of Lyme disease?**

Borrelia burgdorferferi

**What is the causative agent of Lyme disease?**

Borrelia burgdorferi, spread by the Ixodes tick

**What is the most common cranial neuropathy associated with Lyme disease?**

Bell's palsy.

**What is the most common cranial neuropathy seen in patients with Lyme disease?**

Facial nerve neuropathy is most commonly seen, often misdiagnosed as Bell's palsy

**What is the most common neurologic symptom of Lyme disease?**

Headaches, mild stiff neck, and photophobia

**What is the most common ocular manifestation of Lyme disease?**

Conjunctivitis is seen in approximately 11% of patients.

**What is the most common pattern of arthritis associated with Lyme disease?**

Lyme arthritis most commonly presents with an asymmetrical monarthritic or oligoarthritic arthritis

of

**What is the most common tick borne disease in the United States?**

Lyme disease

**What is the most frequent neurologic symptom of early disseminated Lyme disease?**

Cranial neuritis, often manifested as facial palsy

**What type of tick transmits Lyme disease to humans?**

Ixodes tick

**Which joint is most commonly affected in patients with Lyme disease related arthritis?**

The knee joint is most commonly affected.

**Describe the infection with Lymphogranuloma venereum?**

-This STD is caused by a virus.

-The primary lesion on vulva occurs 3-4 days after exposure

-Two to three weeks later, marked inguinal adenitis appears

-Meningitis, pleurisy, peritonitis, arthritis can all develop

**What is the etiology of lymphogranuloma venereum?**

Lymphogranuloma venereum is caused by the L1, L2, and L3 serovars of Chlamydia trachomatis

**What are the 4 types of malaria?**

Plasmodium falciparum

Plasmodium vivax

Plasmodium malariae

Plasmodium ovale

**What type of mosquito is known to transmit the plasmodium protozoan?**

Anopheles mosquito

**How do you treat contacts of patients with Haemophilus influenza meningitis?**

Prophylactic rifampin to treat nasopharyngeal carriers

**What bacteria is the most common infection of central nervous system shunts?**

Staphylococcal epidermidis

**What is the most common cause of bacterial meningitis?**

Streptococcus pneumonia

**What is the bactericidal mechanism of metronidazole?**

Metronidazole forms toxic metabolites in the bacterial cell wall

**What is the warning for patients taking metronidazole?**

Avoid drinking alcohol

**Should patients with mononucleosis avoid contact sports within one month of illness?**

Yes, there is an increased risk of splenic rupture in these patients

**What are seven causes of heterophile negative mononucleosis?**

CMV

HIV-1

Adenovirus

Herpes Simplex II

EBV

Toxoplasma

Rubella

**When is splenomegaly most likely to occur in patients with infectious mononucleosis?**

During the second week of illness

**What are the two fungi that are most often known to cause rhinocerebral mucormycosis?**

Rhizopus and Rhizomucor are the most often causes of rhinocerebral mucormcosis

**What patient population has a specific risk factor for mucormycosis?**

Patients on dialysis who are receiving deferoxamine iron chelation

**What type of cold agglutinins can develop with mycoplasma pneumoniae infections?**

Mycoplasma pneumonia generally is associated with an IgM anti-I

**Which bacteria is most associated with the development of cold agglutinins?**

Mycoplasma pneumonia

**What is the cause of primary amebic meningoencephalitis?**

Naegleria fowleri is the cause of primary amebic meningoencephalitis. It is seen 2-5 days after swimming

**What is the etiology of neurocysticercosis?**

Taenia solium

**What is the most common parasitic disease of the CNS?**

Neurocysticercosis (Taenia solium)

**What is the most common symptom in patients with neurocysticercosis?**

Seizures occur in 70-90% of patients

**Which type of infection can commonly cause overwhelming sepsis in untreated patients with neutropenia?**

Gram negative septicemia

**What is a weakly acid fast, filamentous gram positive organisms?**

Nocardia

**What is the most common clinical manifestation of Nocardia infection?**

Pulmonary infection

**What is the most common Nocardia species to cause human infection in the United States?**

Nocardia asteroides

**What is the most common gram negative organism associated with osteomyelitis?**

E. coli

**What multifocal progressive demyelination of the white matter is associated with Papova virus?**

Progressive multifocal leukoencephalopathy (PML)

**Can pelvic inflammatory disease be the result of a sexually transmitted disease?**

Yes

**How often are men with Neisseria gonorrhea and Chlamydia trachomatis infections asymptomatic?**

Approximately 1/2 of men with gonorrhea and Chlamydia have symptoms

**How often do patients with pelvic inflammatory disease have a recent history of fever?**

Approximately 50% of patients with PID will have a history of a recent fever

**How often does perihepatitis (Fitz-Hugh Curtis syndrome) develop secondary to pelvic inflammatory disease?**

Approximately 10% of women with PID will develop perihepatitis

**How often does PID occur secondary to Chlamydia trachomatis?**

Approximately 33% of PID cases occur secondary to Chlamydia trachomatis

**How often does PID occur secondary to Neisseria gonorrhea?**

Approximately 33% of PID cases occur secondary to Neisseria gonorrhea

**How often will patients with PID have a leukocytosis on the CBC?**

Less than half of patients will have leukocytosis on CBC

**How often will women with Chlamydia trachomatis develop PID?**

Approximately 15% of women with endocervical Chlamydia will develop PID

**How often will women with Neisseria gonorrhea develop PID?**

Approximately 15% of women with endocervical gonorrhea will develop PID

**Is PID more likely to occur around the time of menses?**

As much as 75% of PID occurs within 7 days of menses

**Is there a benefit of using combination therapy with pentamidine and trimethoprim-sulfamethoxazol?**

No, there is no proven added benefit of using the agents in combination

**Who is at the greatest risk of developing Klebsiella pneumonia outside the hospital setting?**

Alcoholics

**What is the most common source of human psittacosis?**

Parrots, parakeets, and budgerigars

**How often will blood cultures be positive in patients with pyelonephritis?**

Blood cultures will return positive in approximately 15-20% of patients diagnosed with pyelonephritis

**What are the common symptoms of pyelonephritis?**

Patients often have fever, dysuria, rigors, flank pain, hematuria, and nausea

**What are the physical exam findings of pyelonephritis?**

Patients with pyelonephritis often have costovertebral tenderness and flank pain

**What are the typical urinary findings in patients with pyelonephritis?**

The urine generally will demonstrate hematuria, pyuria, and leukocyte casts

**What type of bacteria most commonly cause pyelonephritis?**

Gram negative bacteria such as E. coli and Klebsiella spp. are responsible for more than 90% of cases

**What is the most common cause of rabies in the United States?**

The most common cause of rabies in the US is exposure to a dog outside the United States

## What is the ASO test used for?

Rising titers of the ASO test is a sensitive indicator of a previous streptococcal infection

**How soon after an infection with streptococcus would you expect the ASO titers to rise?**

Approximately 1-3 weeks after onset of infection

**How long will it take for the ASO titer to fall after resolution of a streptococcal infection?**

The ASO titer should fall to normal in 6-12 months

**How often should ASO titers be measured when looking for a rise?**

Approximately every 2-3 weeks

**How often will the ASO titer be elevated in patients with post-streptococcal glomerulonephritis?**

Approximately 50% of patients with post-streptococcal glomerulonephritis will have elevated ASO titer

**How often will the ASO titers be elevated in acute rheumatic fever?**

Approximately 80-90% of patients with acute rheumatic fever will have an elevated ASO titer

**How often are rising ASO titers seen in untreated streptococcal pharyngitis infections?**

Approximately 80%

**Will the use of penicillin in patients with streptococcal pharyngitis alter the rise in the ASO titers?**

Yes, penicillin will prevent or decrease the rise of the ASO titers related to streptococcal pharyngitis

**What are the white spots of coagulated fibrin in the retina associated with bacterial endocarditis?**

Roth spots

**Describe the Sabin polio vaccine?**

The Sabin vaccine is given orally and composed of live attenuated polio virus.

**How should salmonella intestinal infection be treated?**

-Supportive therapy only

-No antibiotics should be given unless accompanied by septicemia because antibiotics may prolong infection

-No drugs should be given which slow intestinal motility

**What infection is the cause of San Joaquin Valley fever?**

Coccidioides immitus

**Describe the two stages of septic shock?**

Early- Vasodilatation resulting in warm skin, full pulses, and normal urine output

Late- Vasoconstriction and poor urine outputs, mental status changes, hypotension

**What are two common early signs of sepsis in the elderly?**

Respiratory alkalosis and

Mental confusion

**What is the most common cause of bacterial sepsis associated with purpura fulminans?**

Neisseria meningitis
(meningococcemia)

**What is the most common cause of septic intracranial thrombophlebitis?**

Staphylococcus aureus

**List 4 potential complications of sinusitis?**

Cerebral abscess

Subdural empyema

Cortical thrombophlebitis

Osteomyelitis

**What are 3 common causative organisms of chronic sinusitis?**

Anaerobes (Bacteroides, vionella, rhino bacterium)

**Prior to eradication of smallpox, what were the two strains of the variola virus?**

Variola major (smallpox) and variola minor (alastrim)

**Does smallpox require vectors for spread of disease?**

No, smallpox is directly spread person to person

**How does the smallpox virus most commonly enter the human body?**

It most commonly enters through the respiratory system

**Is smallpox more or less transmissible than chickenpox, measles, and influenza?**

Smallpox is less transmissible than chickenpox, measles, and influenza.

**Is there a way to differentiate monkey pox from smallpox?**

Monkey pox is associated with more lymphadenopathy, but is virtually indistinguishable from smallpox

**Is there any benefit from vaccinating persons exposed to a patient with smallpox?**

Yes, if vaccination to smallpox occurs within 3 days of exposure, there is significant protection

**What are the 5 types of smallpox as classified by the WHO?**

1. Ordinary, 2. Modified, 3. Hemorrhagic, 4. Flat type, 5. Variola sine eruptione

**What is the incubation period of smallpox?**

The incubation period of smallpox is 7-17 days

**What is the virus which causes smallpox?**

The variola virus is known to cause smallpox

**What was the mortality of variola major (smallpox) infection?**

The overall mortality was approximately 20-50%

**What was the mortality of variola minor (alastrim) infection?**

The overall mortality was <1% for the variola minor infection

**When was the last case of endemic smallpox known to occur?**

The last case of endemic smallpox occurred in Somalia in 1977

**Which type of bacteria are most common in post splenectomy patients?**

Encapsulated organisms such as H. influenza and S. pneumoniae

**What is the leading cause of spontaneous bacterial peritonitis?**

E. coli

**What is the most common cause of acute osteomyelitis?**

Staphylococcus aureus

**What is the most common cause of soft tissue and skin infections?**

Staphylococcus aureus

**What is the most common cause of septic intracranial epidural thrombophlebitis?**

Staphylococcus aureus

**What is the most common cause of spinal epidural abscess?**

Staphylococcus aureus

**What is the factor most strongly associated with virulence of streptococcal?**

Streptococcal M protein helps resist against phagocytosis

**What is the most common complication of pneumococcal pneumonia?**

Empyema is the most common complication of pneumococcal pneumonia (2% occurrence)

**What type of bacteria are gram-positive cocci that grow in chains and are catalase negative?**

Streptococcus pneumonia

**Does the FTA-ABS become positive prior to the RPR or VDRL?**

Yes

**How long will the FTA-ABS remain positive after treatment for syphilis?**

Approximately 24% of patients will become sero-negative after 3 years

**What disease is characterized by lymphadenopathy and a papulosquamous rash involving the palms?**

Secondary syphilis

**What is an Argyll-Robertson pupil which is characteristic of tertiary syphilis?**

The pupil constricts with accommodation but is not reactive to light

## What is the FTA-ABS?

The FTA-ABS tests for IgM and IgG antibodies to treponema in patients suspected of having syphilis

**What is the specific predilection of Syphilitic heart disease?**

Tertiary syphilis disrupts the vasa vasorum via obliterative endarteritis and disrupts elastica

**Why the FTA-ABS is most commonly performed?**

To rule out a false positive nontreponenal test for syphilis

**Which antibiotic is bacteriostatic, binds to 30s and prevents the attachment of aminoacyl-tRNA; it is known for its side effect of discoloring teeth?**

Tetracycline

**What is the most common symptom of toxoplasmosis in immunocompetent patients?**

Painless lymphadenopathy

**Which animal is associated with spread of toxoplasmosis?**

Toxoplasmosis can be spread in cat feces

**What is the most common cause of scalp infections in the United States?**

Trichophyton tonsurans

**What are two things that persons taking isoniazid should avoid?**

Alcohol and Acetaminophen

**What is considered positive for TB skin test in patients who are HIV positive?**

Induration > 5mm

**What is the most common clinical form of tuberculosis?**

Reactivation tuberculosis is the most common clinical form of TB

**What is the most common location for post-primary TB?**

Apical and posterior segments of upper lobes (85%)

**What is the standard 4 drug therapy for TB?**

-Isoniazid

-Pyrazinamide

-Rifampin

Ethambutol

**Which infection is suggested by an exudative pleural fluid with >90% lymphocytes?**

Tuberculosis

**What are the attenuated live bacterial vaccines?**

Typhoid

BCG

**What are the attenuated live virus vaccines?**

Mumps-measles-rubella (MMR)

Oral Polio

Yellow fever

**What are the dead bacterial vaccines?**

Cholera

H. Influenza

Pneumococcal

Typhoid

Meningococcal

**What are the dead virus vaccines?**

Injectable polio

Hepatitis A

Hepatitis B

Rabies

Influenza

**What is the group of bacteria covered commonly with vancomycin?**

Gram positive bacteria

**What is the mechanism of Vancomycin?**

Vancomycin inhibits cell wall mucopeptide formation

**Are birds more likely to be infected with the West Nile Virus than humans?**

Yes

**Is there any specific treatment for the West Nile Virus?**

No, at this time there is no specific treatment. Supportive care is the standard.

**The West Nile Virus is an arbovirus, what does the term arbovirus mean?**

Arbovirus is short for "arthropod-borne-virus"

**What is the incubation period in humans for the West Nile Virus?**

The incubation period for the West Nile Virus is 3-15 days

**What is the primary reservoir for the West Nile Virus?**

Infected birds are the main reservoir for the West Nile Virus

**When was the first outbreak of the West Nile Virus in the United States?**

The first outbreak of the West Nile Virus was in New York in the summer of 1999

**Where did the West Nile Virus name originate?**

West Nile Virus was initially isolated in an infected woman in the West Nile district of Uganda in 1937

The rash of zoster is described as an erythematous maculaopapular rash progressing to clusters of clear vesicles.

Anti-HBc is the earliest indication of an acute hepatitis B infection.

The presence of HBsAg indicates an acute or chronic infection with hepatitis B.

A person with chickenpox (varicella) can spread chickenpox, but cannot spread shingles. Shingles only occurs when there is a reactivation of a latent infection.

Anti-Hbe indicates resolution of an acute infection with hepatitis B.

Anti-HBs indicates the presence of immunity to hepatitis B either from a previous infection or vaccination.

Blood cultures will return positive in approximately 15-20% of patients diagnosed with pyelonephritis.

Among patients with normal immune system, post herpetic neuralgia develops in about 10% of patients.

Lung abscesses are most likely to be found in the posterior segments of the upper lobes and the apical segments of the lower lobes. These areas are dependent when the patient is recumbent.

The urine in patients with pyelonephritis generally will demonstrate hematuria, pyuria, and leukocyte casts

Exposure to a person with shingles can result in chickenpox in another person who is not immune to the varicella virus.

Further workup (CT scan, IVP, or renal ultrasound) should be done to rule out abscess or stone in patients with pyelonephritis who do not have improvement in their symptoms after given antibiotics for 48 hours.

The symptoms of the West Nile virus are nonspecific. These include fever, headache, myalgias, neck pain, weakness, vomiting, photophobia, mental status changes, and diarrhea.

Typical cerebrospinal fluid (CSF) findings in patients with CNS involvement of the West Nile virus reveal <100 wbc/mm3 with a lymphocytic pleocytosis associated with an elevated CSF protein concentration.

Acute hepatitis B can be characterized by an elevated ALT and development of Anti HBc.

Shingles most commonly occurs on the thorax.

Streptococcus pneumoniae are gram-positive cocci that grow in chains and are catalase negative.

Approximately 33% of new HSV-2 infections are symptomatic.

HSV-2 is responsible for 70-95% of the genital herpes infections.

Approximately 2% of nursing mothers will develop mastoiditis, and approximately 6-7% of those women will develop a breast abscess.

Brucellosis is a zoonotic infection most commonly caused by a gram negative coccobacillus, Brucella melitensis. It generally occurs after animal exposure and often presents as a febrile illness.

Aspirin is associated with an increased incidence of Reye's syndrome. Fever and myalgias in children should be treated with acetaminophen as appropriate.

Several other diseases are seen more often in patients with hepatitis C including but not limited to glomerulonephritis, porphyria cutanea tarda, cryoglobulinemia, polyarthritis, and monoclonal gammopathy.

Chronic hepatitis B is characterized by the presence of HBsAg for more than 6 months without the development of detectable anti-HBs antibody.

The classic triad of patients presenting with a brain abscess:- Headache; Fever; Focal neurological deficits.

Sometimes patients can have a less severe infection with HSV-2 if they have been previously exposed to HSV-1.

Sickle cell disease, asplenia, and agammaglobulinemia predispose to infections with encapsulated organisms.

Genital herpes infection generally develops approximately 2-7 days after exposure and is associated with fever, malaise, inguinal adenopathy and vesicular lesions in the genital region.

Recurrence of herpes simplex 1 is associated with trauma, cold, sunlight, stress, wind, menstruation, and fever.

EBV has been associated with
Burkitt's lymphoma and
nasopharyngeal carcinoma.

It is possible for HSV-1 to infect the genital region and HSV-2 to infect the mouth and perioral region.

It is thought that sporadic Listeria infection can occur after ingestion of unpasteurized or contaminated milk, soft cheeses, and meat.

A ghon complex is the TB granulomas with lobar or perihilar lymph node involvement.

Fact: The primary varicella infection presents as chicken pox. A reactivation of varicella-zoster in the dorsal root ganglia can present as the shingles.

Patients with infectious mononucleosis can develop hemolytic anemia related to development of an autoantibody to the "i" antigen on the red cells.

Approximately 50% of the population in the US has serologic evidence of exposure to the Epstein Barr Virus by 5 y/o.

Infants with granulomatosis infantiseptica from severe trans placental Listeria infection generally have internal organs with multiple granulomas or abscesses associated with papular or ulcerative skin lesions.

Listeria is the most common cause of bacterial meningitis in patients with cancer, particularly those who have lymphoma, those who have had a bone marrow transplant, or those who are receiving corticosteroids.

The Salk vaccine is inactivated and given via injection. It does not provide lifelong immunity to polio and requires periodic booster shots.

Approximately 20-40% of primary herpes simplex 1 infections of the lips or perioral regions will recur.

The Sabin vaccine is given orally and composed of live attenuated polio virus. This vaccine provides lifelong immunity.

The West Nile Virus is most closely related to the virus isolated from a dead goose in Israel in 1998. It is thought that the virus was transmitted by infected birds or mosquitoes to the New York airport from the Middle East.

Approximately 1/3 of patients with bacterial endocarditis will develop neurologic symptoms. These are characterized by cerebral emboli (20% of patients) and encephalopathy (10% of patients).

About 50% of college age persons who seroconvert after exposure to the Epstein Barr virus will developed infectious mononucleosis.

Approximately 10% of people with infectious mononucleosis will develop a maculopapular diffuse rash. This is seen more commonly in people given ampicillin.

Mammals are dead end vectors of the West Nile virus because mosquitoes can bite infected humans or horses and not pick up the virus due to low viral loads.

Most people infected with the West Nile virus will not become ill. About 30% of infected people will develop a mild flu-like illness, and approximately 1% will develop encephalitis.

The Culex species of the mosquito is the primary vector for West Nile virus.  Other species of mosquitoes known to be vectors include Aedes and the Aenopheles species.

Although birds are the main reservoir of the West Nile virus, fatal infections from West Nile virus have been seen in a cat, skunk, squirrel, rabbit, chipmunk, and bats.

The rash of smallpox is characterized by small reddish macules which develop into 2-3 mm papules, then 2-5 mm vesicles, then 4-6 mm pustules, followed by crusting. These occur on the face and extremities first but progress to cover the whole body.

Viral encephalitis is characterized by pleomorphic lymphocytosis of CSF, no bacteria on gram stain, normal glucose, and negative cultures

Approximately 6 weeks after developing infection with HCV approximately 70% of patients with hepatitis C infection will have anti HCV, and at 6 months approximately 90% will have anti HCV.

In patients with ascaris lumbricoides the peripheral blood eosinophilia is most commonly seen soon after the ingestion of the eggs and development of the larva. Eosinophilia is less common once the adult worms are present.

This concludes Infectious Disease Study Guide: Fast Focus Study Guide

Search Amazon Kindle books to find other study guides written by

JT Thomas, MD

Internal Medicine Study Guide

Medical Oncology Study Guide

Multiple Myeloma Study Guide

Differential Diagnosis Study Guide

Rheumatology Study Guide

www.ingramcontent.com/pod-product-compliance
Lightning Source LLC
Chambersburg PA
CBHW051849170526
45168CB00001B/30
*9781512343304*